ALLISON GRUBER

Themes for Yoga Teachers

A guide for yoga teachers to add meditations, quotes, and yoga themes to their class experience

Contents

Introduction

Welcome to Themes For Yoga Teachers. My name is Ali Gruber and I am extremely excited to be writing this book. As a student of yoga, a teacher of yoga, and a yoga teacher trainer I have seen teachers create incredible alignment-based flow classes, but something still fell short. This is because the true teachings of yoga are much deeper than the physical postures alone. I believe classes that solely focus on asana are missing a huge aspect of what yoga can truly offer our students. As teachers, weaving themes into our classes helps our students experience the richness of yoga, assists them in getting deeper into their practice, and sets the stage for our students to tap into the vast and beautiful world of yoga.

A brief background of myself. I am a forever student who loves to always be learning and love when the topic of my studies is yoga. I took my first yoga class in the winter of 2011 and instantly fell in love. At that time I couldn't articulate exactly why I was feeling incredible and why it was so different from any other fitness classes I took, but I knew I needed to learn more. I signed up for my first Yoga Teacher Training shortly thereafter and graduated in March of 2012. I auditioned and started teaching in a studio one week after graduating with my RYT-200. I continued to learn more about the practice with specialty certificates in Yin Yoga, Prenatal, further training in the Ashtanga lineage, and Power Yoga. I ventured into deepening my understanding of yoga and teaching skills when I completed my RYT-500 training in 2017. I am forever grateful for my teachers and the lineage I have learned from.

This book will give you the ability to transform your teaching by easily theming your yoga classes. Just like building your flows, such as determining where you will put in your sun salutations, what variation of sun salutations, or what your peak pose will be, theming your class is something that demands practice before it becomes second nature. You can now focus on building your flows and allow this guide to help inspire your themes. Please note: having a theme in your class is so much more than simply reading a beautiful quote at the end of your class. Weaving your theme into little nuggets throughout your teachings will help that same beautiful quote you wish to read at the end of your class land so much deeper.

Whether you are new to teaching yoga, feeling uninspired, or just don't have the bandwidth to create a theme for your class you can use this book as a quick tool to help you prepare to deliver a wonderful class experience for your students. I provide theme-based quotes, nuggets of wisdom, example poses, and short meditations or stories that can be woven into your teaching to leave your students feeling layers deeper than the physical practice.

I am looking forward to hearing how you are creating experiences for your students and how they then take these nuggets of information and spread them throughout their lives. Many of these themes can be woven within each other and have overlap, feel free to utilize this as a starting point to create your class talking points. I encourage you to use this book as a place to get inspiration, determine what resonates with you, and incorporate it how you would like within your teaching. After all, our students are going to be different and we are different, what works for me might not work the same for you - and as always, I encourage you to be authentic in your delivery. If a quote or a meditation doesn't sound like something you would say - don't say it! Adapt to work for you, I promise your students will be able to tell the difference!

Let's Dive In!

1

Surrender

Letting Go

In yoga, the practice of letting go can take many forms. It is a simple phrase with a potentially complicated execution. Even for the most advanced yoga practitioners letting go of ego, distractions, expectations, and even senses can be a challenge. Thus, this theme is appropriate for the first-time practitioner and those who have been practicing asana for decades.

You can guide your students to let go of a specific topic or to let go in general. For example, to be specific you could ask your students to let go of a pose looking a certain way or an expectation of how a pose "should" feel. Simply ask your students to observe if they are craving a specific feeling and advise them to release that need to allow a pose to just feel as it is. Are you offering an inversion as an example? Do you have a challenging peak pose? That could be a powerful place to drop a nugget of information inviting them to let go of it looking a specific way (while keeping them safe with proper alignment of course).

Common relatable topics you could incorporate into this theme. Letting go of:

- Mental anxieties
- Attachment to a specific pose
- Anything that is no longer serving you
- Striving for perfection
- Negative thoughts
- Resistance to change
- Comparisons

I love to weave a theme into practice by asking simple questions while teaching. For example, if you are offering a challenging inversion you could ask your students if they really need that inversion right now, or if it's just how they always move. Did that play out how you expected? Whether or not that hard pose worked how you expected or not, does not have any bearing on the success of your practice. Let go of expectations and embrace how you feel right now.

Another way to incorporate letting go is to ask them to let go of tension and draw awareness to their physical body in specific poses. In Warrior 2 remind them to let go of tension in their shoulders or in Childs Pose to let go of clenching their jaws.

Letting Go Quotes

"Some of us think holding on makes us strong but sometimes it is letting go." Hermann Hesse

"Letting go gives us freedom, and freedom is the only condition for happiness." Tich Nhat Hanh

"Becoming the best version of yourself comes with a lot of goodbyes"
Unknown

"You can only lose what you cling to." Buddha

Letting Go Tale

I have told this story in my classes before and always get feedback on how it made students think and feel.

There is a quick story about how monkey catchers trap monkeys in the wild. Catchers place a jar of peanuts on the inside of a small crate. This crate has openings big enough for the monkey's arm to fit through, and the jar that holds the peanut is big enough for the monkey's hand. The monkeys willingly and eagerly slide their arm through the crate and their hand into the jar to grab hold of the peanuts, but when they do their hand gets stuck as they are holding on and grasping too many peanuts. Thus the monkey gets caught easily and with minimal effort from the catcher.

If the monkey would simply let go of the peanuts they could easily slip away from the catcher but the monkey's greed and attachment to peanuts bound them to the jar.

What are your peanuts? What is providing you with a trapped feeling, what can you work to release? After all, aren't we all like the caught monkey at some point or another in our lives?

Acceptance

A central theme in yoga philosophy is acceptance. Finding contentment, loving yourself, caring for yourself, and finding peace are all aspects of acceptance. Yoga asks you to accept who you are, where you are, and to find contentment. The ability to surrender to all of life's comings and goings plays a huge role in overall acceptance.

To accept things as they are or to accept who you are can be hard for people who are always seeking the next best thing or those who never feel as though they are enough. Encourage your students to truly embrace being a "human being" and not a "human doing" through self-acceptance. Part of accepting is truly embracing all the sides of us, the good, the bad, the messy, and everything in between. You can simply invite your students to breathe in anything they need in that moment and lengthen out their exhale, let them know all is welcome and to come as they are, no need to change, and no need to remove what doesn't serve them - that's accepted too.

Acceptance Quote

"Anger is easy, it is one-sided. Acceptance is hard, it requires all sides of you." Unknown

"Yoga is not about self-improvement, you are whole as you are, it is about self-acceptance." Unknown

"Notice the sensation, try to lean into it, fight the need to fight it, and meet it with kindness and acceptance." Me

"I am willing to accept this moment exactly as it is." Unknown

Acceptance Meditation

Bring your awareness to your breath as you settle in. It's ok to experience challenges or to even have awareness of them. Bring something to your mind that feels difficult to accept. It could be an emotion, a situation, or perhaps a part of yourself. As you breathe and focus on this, remind yourself that acceptance does not mean resignation. It's a simple acknowledgment of what is true in this very moment and its reality as is, without clinging to how you wish it to be. Just be.

2

Heart-Opening

Compassion

Compassion is often considered a soft skill yet through the lens of science, studies show that compassion matters not only in meaningful ways but also in measurable ways. We can not give to others what we do not give to ourselves first. The practice of self-compassion in yoga shows up in numerous ways. It can be easy to be hard on ourselves, but when we forgive ourselves, accept our perceived flaws, and offer ourselves kindness we are practicing compassion.

The yoga of self-compassion can be as simple as showing up for yourself and honoring exactly what you need for that specific practice. Guide your students to take a few deep breaths before you introduce movement, the simple act of grounding and bringing awareness inward can allow individuals a moment to check in, and oftentimes this is the first mindful moment of their day. Invite students to allow loving compassion to flow through each and every breath and to carry this intention throughout their practice.

I like to bring compassion back into the fold during challenging poses, asking your students if they are approaching the physical challenge with compassion or ego. Bring them back to self and give them permission to modify, find a suitable variation, or advance a pose based on what they need at that moment.

You will likely find the theme of compassion woven throughout books in your yoga library, even in the Yoga Sutra of Patanjali the importance of compassion for those who are suffering is a key element of living a yogic lifestyle.

Compassion Quotes

"More smiling, less worrying. More compassion, less judgment. More blessed, less stressed. More love, less hate." Roy T. Bennett

"If you want others to be happy, practice compassion. If you want to be happy, practice compassion." Dalai Lama

"By cultivating attitudes of friendliness toward the happy, compassion for the unhappy, delight in the virtuous, and disregard toward the wicked, the mind-stuff retains its undisturbed calmness." The Yoga Sutras

Compassion Meditation

Envision someone in your life, someone you care about and love who may be struggling - a friend, family member, even a stranger if no one comes to mind quickly. Picture their face and imagine a soft glowing light around them. This light represents your compassion for this individual and what they are facing, your understanding, and your love.

As you continue to relax into your breath imagine this light expanding and wrapping around this person, gently embracing them with every single breath. Offering comfort with a traditional loving kindness mantra, "May you be happy. May you be healthy. May you live your life with ease." Repeat this mantra as many times as needed.

Next, expand this feeling of compassion. Allow it to include yourself. Picture this beautiful glowing energetic light surrounding you in warmth and kindness. Fill your heart with this self-love as you silently repeat to yourself, "I am worthy of love and kindness."

Non-judgment

It is human nature to make judgments, what ends up being harmful is when we hold onto these judgments and keep them as our truths. Practicing non-judgment is critical to a yoga lifestyle and can be incorporated into classes in several ways.

Non-judgment in thoughts is a powerful way to get your students to ground into the present moment. This simple practice can help students prepare for larger observations. When we are focused on judgments it is very challenging to hold space to observe and observances are critical to staying present. I like to invite my students to observe their internal monologue. What are you saying to yourself? Do you speak to yourself the way you would speak to your best friend? Are you putting harsh expectations on yourself? Asking a few questions can help your students realize their tendencies which can help lead to personal growth both on and off the yoga mat.

Being non-judgmental is a mindfulness practice. An easy way to bring this to a yoga practice on the mat is to not judge your physical capabilities as you move from pose to pose. Are your front splits pose not to the ground? Cool! Do you barely lift your hips off the ground in bridge pose? No biggie! Do you need to keep your floating toe down on the ground in tree pose? All good!

Being non-judgmental off the mat can also be very beneficial. Non-judgment in thought is a theme you could weave in and out of your classes over and over. Pairing thoughts with the ability to re frame can be a way to take your non-judgment theme further. Not only should you be non-judgmental but you can also re frame the way you think to give more compassion to those we encounter in our lives, including ourselves.

Non Judgment Quotes

"Walking through life with a non-judgmental stance does not render you timid, disappointed, or weak. It helps you sift out the helpful from the harmful, the safe from the dangerous, and effective from the distraction. Non-judgment does not take your power away. It brings it back." Instagram @therapist_in_nyc

"Mindfulness means moment-to-moment, non-judgmental awareness. It is cultivated by refining our capacity to pay attention, intentionally, in the present moment, and then sustaining that attention over time as best we can. In the process, we become more in touch with our life as it is unfolding." Jon Kabat-Zinn

Non-Judgment Tale

There are many yoga stories on non-judgments but one you will likely hear over and over is on the lotus flower. The metaphor of a lotus flower to a human experience is how the lotus grows in muddy and mucky water yet it blooms beautifully. Humans are similar in that we might have to grow over, around, and through the mud that comes our way, and through this "mud" we can grow beautifully. Not judging the mud can be helpful in our growth. If you share a story about the lotus flower I highly recommend incorporating the "No Mud, No Lotus" quote at some point in your class.

3

Pose Based Themes

Utkatasana, Chair Pose, Strength

Many students have a strong feeling about chair pose, and often it's a negative one, but it is a massive strength builder that is accessible to many students. It is a staple in a traditional Surya Namaskar B, and often is utilized as an edge pose and embodies building strength. Chair pose is a muscular pose that can be found in many sequences.

When theming around a specific pose, I like to foreshadow the pose in my warm-up with a focus on the specific muscle groups that will be required to activate in order to hold the specific shape later in practice. For chair pose, I make sure my students have the chance to experience awareness of their legs including ankles, calves, thighs, quadriceps, and hamstrings. This helps them to stabilize their chair pose. In addition, I would spend some time strengthening their core and twisting their spine before the first chair pose.

Teaching challenging and muscularly tough poses can be a great way to remind your students to embrace the challenges and to appreciate what they can do versus focusing on what they can't do. Remind students of how strong they are, even if they fall out of a pose. Remind them that they can do tough things. Remind them that staying in a pose doesn't define their practice. Remind them that holding a pose doesn't define success. Give them space to trust their body and come out if they need to, while also giving them space to explore further. Here are some options to deepen your chair pose.

Variations of Chair Pose:

- Revolved chair pose with prayer hands
- Revolved chair pose with open arms (upright or top arm high, bottom arm low)
- Chair pose with airplane arms
- Chair pose with airplane arms and heels lifted
- Figure four chair pose

Quotes on building strength

"This pose doesn't have to look dramatic to feel dramatic, it is harder than you might think." Me

"Do not judge me by my successes - judge me by how many times I fell down and got back up again." Nelson Mandela

"We don't even know how strong we are until we are forced to bring that hidden strength forward." Isabel Allende

"Never forget how far you've come. Everything you have gotten through.

All the times you have pushed on even when you felt you couldn't. All the mornings you got out of bed no matter how hard it was. All the times you wanted to give up but you got through another day. Never forget how much strength you have developed along the way" Power of Positivity

Hanumanasana, Splits Pose, Flexibility

I have seen students, over and over, feel successful and powerful when they achieve their full front splits pose and on the flip side, feel defeated when they cannot get down to the ground. Hanumanasana or splits pose is a powerful pose to have as your peak and to bring in the theme of flexibility.

Preparing the body for front splits pose can be incorporated into your warm-up poses, first flows, and even in holds such as a standing forward fold. I love to think of this pose as a complete progression; starting with shapes like a supine hamstring stretch with or without the addition of a yoga strap, a forward fold hold, a half splits pose with different variations, a pyramid pose, and dynamic ways of moving in and out of stretching the hamstrings to support front splits. When a student is properly warmed up, and a grand finale pose arises, they are prepared to explore the depth of the intended pose that feels best for their body that day.

Teaching your students that flexibility is not only represented in our physical body but also in our thoughts and mind can help them tremendously. Remind your students to approach their practice with a flexible mind and not to hold onto a rigid pattern of thinking. This can help them explore new depths in their practice.

Advancements and other variation examples:

- Standing splits
- Over splits
- Super soldier
- Flying splits

Quotes on flexibility

"Nothing is softer or more flexible than water, yet nothing can resist it."
Lao Tzu

"Stay committed to your decisions, but stay flexible in your approach."
Tony Robbins

"Flexibility is the key to stability" John Wooden

Be Flexible: A lesson from Aesop

An oak and a reed were arguing about their strength. When a strong wind came up, the reed avoided being uprooted by bending and leaning with the gusts of wind. But the oak stood firm and was torn up by the roots. This simple story reminds us to be flexible in order to remain strong and resilient.

If you choose to do a pose-based theme find what resonates and stick with it, otherwise, your strong teachings might get lost in your pose teaching!

4

Chakra

Root Chakra

All of the Chakras can be incorporated into a class theme and can give your students a beautiful way to understand the power of our subtle body. Our Root Chakra, Muladhara Chakra, or often referenced as our first Chakra is located at the base of the spine, think of your tailbone and think of the color red. It is the first of seven Chakras associated with our body.

Our Root Chakra is responsible for our sense of security, feeling stable, and grounding in our lives. Alignment in our Root Chakra helps us feel balanced and happy, it also assists in removing anxieties in our lives.

A practice that is focused on the Root Chakra would typically focus on grounding postures with an emphasis on the lower body. Many of the poses associated with a Root Chakra practice are often ones that can be enough with just a small amount of sensation. They don't need to be these huge massive and exhilarating postures. This Chakra is rooted in our basic needs, it doesn't need to be fancy, it just needs to feel grounded.

Here is a sample list of Root Chakra poses:

- Child's pose
- Happy baby
- Forward fold
- Malasana
- Seated butterfly
- Seated wide leg forward fold
- Seated meditation
- Supported bridge
- Savasana

Quotes on being grounded

"Stay humble, stay grounded, remember what got you to that level - and that's hard work." Tim Howard

"When adversity strikes, that's when you have to be the most calm. Take a step back, stay strong, stay grounded and press on." LL Cool J

Root Chakra affirmations:

- I am grounded
- I am secure
- I am safe
- I have enough
- I am enough
- The universe provides all I need

- I can handle anything that comes my way
- I feel connected to the earth and its supportive energy

Note on incorporating Chakras: You can have an entire class centered on a Chakra without ever even saying the word Chakra. Depending on your students, utilizing Sanskrit words or incorporating details on philosophy can sometimes leave them confused. Keep it simple and explain things how you would simply explain to someone you were sharing a meal with! There is a tremendous amount of beauty in simplicity.

Heart Chakra

Our Heart Chakra, Anahata Chakra, often referred to as our fourth Chakra is located at our heart center right in the center of your chest behind your sternum. Our Heart Chakra is responsible for our ability to love and to be loved. It is often associated with balance, calmness, and serenity. Alignment with our Heart Chakra helps us stay connected in compassion for ourselves and for others.

A practice that is focused on the Heart Chakra would typically focus on backbends and the upper back. These types of poses are quite literally exposing our heart center and help us to breathe more freely. In addition, Bhakti yoga, or the yoga of devotion, is heavily connected to Anahata Chakra. One powerful way to weave this theme into your practice is to talk about the benefits of an aligned Heart Chakra while your students are holding a bridge pose or another heart opener.

Here is a sample list of Heart Chakra poses:

- Supported fish

- Melting heart/puppy pose
- Bridge
- Full wheel

Quotes on opening your heart

"In a world where you can open any door, first of all, choose to open the door of your heart." Alexandra V

"You can't always protect your heart, sometimes the only way to be safe is to open it."

Heart Chakra affirmations

- I can forgive myself and others
- I deserve love
- I deserve to be loved
- I love myself without any further conditions
- I am loved and am worthy
- I can give and receive joy

A powerful way to incorporate a Heart Chakra affirmation is to have your students settle into a seated meditation and place one or both hands over their hearts, ask them to close their eyes, and silently repeat an affirmation after you.

5

Yoga Sutra

Yoga Sutra 1.2

The Yoga Sutras hold a world of incredible information to share with your clients. Traditionally, students of yoga are intended to sit with one Sutra at a time and truly absorb its meaning before continuing to study, our students don't need to approach the learning that come from the Sutras in the same way that a teacher might approach studying this topic.

One of my favorite Yoga Sutras to theme in a practice is Yoga Sutra 1.2. This Sutra says "Yogas chitta vritti nirodha." This is translated into multiple different variations of sayings with the same general meaning, including the following:

- The restraint of the modifications of the mind stuff
- Cessations of the fluctuations of the mind
- Cessations of the misidentification with the modifications of the mind

- Calming the monkey mind

This Sutra teaches us that clearing our mind is an important step in yoga, it's so important it even comes before any physical movement. I love to incorporate words such as clear, concentration, and presence when incorporating this Sutra into my themes.

Quotes related to Yoga Sutra 1.2

"Watch your thoughts, they become your words; watch your words, they become your actions; watch your actions, they become your habits; watch your habits, they become your character; watch your character, it becomes your destiny." Lao Tzu

"Your calm mind is the ultimate weapon against challenges." Bryant McGill

"The mind is like water. When it's turbulent, it's difficult to see. When it's calm, everything becomes clear." Buddha

Here is an example of utilizing Yoga Sutra 1.2 in your class:

- Start of class: "Notice your breath, start to lengthen out your exhales, and give more time to empty out completely. Notice the rise of your belly as you breathe in this incredible life force. Notice the sensations that arise. Often a very simple slowing of our breath can help to clear our mind. Allow thoughts that arise to have their movement and then simply let them know. Using this time to calm our mind as we begin to move."
- During your flow: "Notice if your thoughts have drifted, bring it back to your breath and movement."

- During your peak pose: "Clear your mind of can't. Calm mind, calm breath, and go give it a shot, give it your all."
- End of class: "Remaining calm in every situation helps your mind find solutions. Calmness reflects trust and instead of overthinking or reacting impulsively, you surrender in the moment, opening yourself to guidance and clarity for what may seem unclear."

6

Additional Themes & Considerations

This is by no means an exhaustive list, just a result of brainstorming topics to get your creative juices flowing.

- Turning inward
- Quit your mind
- Balance effort and ease
- Moving meditation
- Yamas
- Niyamas
- You are enough as is
- Gratitude
- Open to change
- Listen to your body
- Find balance
- Beginner mindset
- Be curious
- Practice forgiveness
- Practice, not perfection

- Embrace discomfort
- Trust yourself

This list could go on and on! I encourage you to teach themes that resonate with you. Speaking of, continue on for a few more tips.

Tips for Theming Your Yoga Class

Please please please don't harp on a theme or overdo it. Keep it simple and give space for the theme to settle in your students the way that resonates with them. Try to stay away from repeating Sanskrit terms and try to utilize normal language that you use in your teaching, that being said, if you are teaching in a Sanskrit heavy studio then by all means, your students will be used to it!

Try to keep lengthy personal stories out of it. I was in a class that had an entire meditation based on the feeling of visiting your grandparents, which is beautiful, however, it was the only visualization offered to try to get students to a specific feeling. You might think this is fine, but what if your student just recently lost a grandparent? Just something to consider.

Don't miss opportunities to include little nuggets throughout your class. If the only time you are bringing in your inspirational talk is with a quote at the end of the class you are missing so many chances to impact your student's lives and this is truly not theming your class. One tip that helped me out with my own teaching was to use a notebook while teaching. In an open notebook, I write my flow on the right page and write the nuggets, quotes, and meditations on the left page to ensure I don't forget any nuggets.

Be authentic, always. If a theme doesn't sit well with you, don't teach it! There are so many incredible options and theme possibilities out there.

7

Conclusion

There are unlimited ways to theme your classes and to bring important yoga philosophies to your teaching skills. What you authentically bring to your students will shape the way they feel about yoga and ultimately keep them coming back to your class. I hope you enjoyed reading this book as much as I enjoyed writing it.

If you found this book helpful I would be very grateful if you left a favorable review on Amazon. A little kind word would go a long way.

Thank you!

Resources

Be flexible: A lesson from Aesop. (2006). In *Strengthening Family Resilience*. The Guilford Press. https://blogs.extension.wisc.edu/co -parenting/files/2014/12/FR-2BeFlexible.pdf

Bennett, R. T. (2020). *The light in the heart: Inspirational Thoughts for Living Your Best Life*. Sweatt, L. (2024, September 25). *50 Quotes about Strength: Words to boost your inner power*. SUCCESS. https://www.suc cess.com/21-motivational-quotes-about-strength/

Trzeciak, S., Mazzarelli, A., & Seppälä, E. (2023, March 2). *Leading with Compassion Has Research-Backed Benefits*. Harvard Business Review. https://hbr.org/2023/02/leading-with-compassion-has-research-back ed-benefits

Vivekananda, S. (2024). *Patanjali Yoga Sutra: Patanjali Yoga Sutra: Swami Vivekananda's Insights into the Path of Yoga (Namasakr Books)*. Namasakr Books.

Xiv, D. L., Bstan-'dzin-Rgya-Mtsho, D. L. X., & Cutler, H. C. (2009). *The art of happiness: A Handbook for Living*.

* 9 7 9 8 3 0 0 4 0 8 7 8 7 *